Running Low and Slow:
Winning the Race from Last Place
700 Meters to Marathon in 9 Months

Daria Yadernaya

CONTENTS

ACKNOWLEDGMENTS

I'm devoting these pages to people who encouraged me when I started running and stood by me at all times.

To the Moscow Road Runners club whose Whatsapps motivate me to get my butt out of bed and put on sneakers every time.

To Masha Kurdina, who got this crazy idea of us running in Nice, France.

To my coach Alexey Vorobiev who always knew I could and gave me all the overall and interval training I needed to become a healthy runner.

and last but not the least to my fiancé, Rob Brown who survived many unpleasant moments when I was running, and after I ran.

INTRODUCTION

Running is fun, they will tell you. When you start running, it's never fun, unless you were an athlete in your previous life. Running is sweat, exhaustion and longing to stop with every step. They will promise you it will get better and it won't. At first.

So many people give up after starting to run, and for a good reason. It's too difficult, too tiring and too painful. All this might be true; but the truth is, it's the most natural exercise, the most affordable, complex, invigorating, and fun. Yet you have to work to get to the point where it actually is fun. And sometimes trying to get motivated by all those great runners we follow on social media just doesn't work for a simple reason – you are not them.

Their paces are too fast, their distances are too long, they are too fit and too healthy and their eating habits are too perfect. You are a regular person, with your own complexities and a multitude of layers of personality. You eat garbage sometimes (probably many times), you don't exercise regularly and your life isn't devoted to sports, you don't move around much, you get stressed and you don't sleep enough sometimes. You are human, and all these people seem too distant and too ideal to you.

In this book I'm writing about people like you and me, the regular people. People who are not super fit, or ideal, or healthy. We are the people who just lead a regular life of their own and are trying to incorporate some healthy habits into their lifestyle. Why not start with running? And most importantly, how not to give up running and start enjoying it; for life and pleasure, and health of course.

I'm writing for those who don't feel like running as they feel ashamed of themselves, of the fact that people will be staring or disapproving. People who don't take part in races as they are terrified to run to the very end and to finish last, or not finish at all. I'm writing for somebody who is just like me, a concealed champion, who wins from the inside and comes last in races, and thinks that's okay too.

So let's get started!

1 WHY DO WE RUN?

So why do we run? A quick survey among my friends showed various reasons.

1. It's fashionable
2. Everybody runs around me, it's part of the social culture
3. I want to lose weight
4. It's an easy-to-do-everywhere workout
5. It's fun
6. It helps me make friends
7. It helps me calm down
8. I like running races

Interesting, how many different the reasons there might be for running. They might combine both personal reasons of being healthy and having fun to social reasons like being trendy or mixing with the right people. In fact, it does matter why you run. Depending on how ambitious you get about running you will chose a different approach to running.

More ambitious people set higher targets of taking part in races, prepping for a half-marathon, a marathon and even an ultra-marathon. Some take a more balanced approach to running, such as just enough to stay in shape and being among the right social group. Some run regularly, others opt for occasional socially important runs, such as charity or corporate races. Depending on why you run you might encounter different problems, some of them psychological which might push you to quit.

Reasons for running and problems they create

Reasons	Problems
It's fashionable	You don't know how to run and how much you should run, so overtraining and injuries are possible when you try to keep up with more "advanced" friends.
Everybody runs around me, it's part of the social culture	
I want to lose weight	Losing weight is one of the consequences of

	running, but not a guaranteed one. A balanced eating regime is required as well as general fitness workouts. By the way, the more you run, the faster your metabolism, so you might actually be wanting to eat more – thus, not really lose weight. Besides, weight is not an indicator, muscle to fat ratio is, and working on it is a completely different story.
It's an easy-to-do-everywhere workout	That one is true, but beware of different weather conditions if you travel, different surface and living conditions such as air and water. You also have to think about the surface and different shoes that might be required, and different sports gear, so it might not be that easy.

It's fun	Well, that depends. I had been running for 5 months before I started enjoying it, and that's with running 5 times a week to prep for races, and running a beautiful race in Nice, France.
It helps me make friends	That is definitely true, however that might mean you have to keep up with fitter and better prepared friends, which sometimes makes you feel depressed that you cannot reach their level right away.
It helps me calm down	That one is true – once you are fit enough to actually enjoy running and divert your thoughts away from the actually process and pains of running.
I like running races	Only if you are good runner, you might think. And this is fundamentally wrong. In this book I'll

	try to target the approach for winning the race by just finishing it, irrespective of what the ranking says at the end.

So, for whatever reason you run you might find barriers that try to prevent you from becoming a runner, and the most fundamental of them is, you might not be as good at it as you expected. You might not be as fast as you wanted. You might not be able to run as far as you thought you would. You might not be able to get as fit as you wanted, and people around you might be expecting more from you. Or, at least, that's what you think. Those are the most essential barriers, and they are all in your mind. So let's try and fight them.

2 HOW DO WE RUN?

How do we normally start running? Looking at the social media, it seems very easy to go and run 5 kilometers, as many of our friends and acquaintances and people we are watching on Facebook and Instagram easily knock out 10 km runs. So you think 5 is a minimum. And here is your first delusion. 5 kilometers is a lot.

My first runs were 700 meters, which is less than half a mile. It was one lap around the pond in the park where I had workouts with my coach. I swear there was never, ever any longer distance than this freaking pond in my whole life. By the way, I ran two marathons after that.

My coach would sit on the bench on the edge of the pond and watch me run. There was a small restaurant at the far side of the pond, that blocked like around 100 meters of the route from his view. So he could watch me run the whole way except for this one, small blind spot. So guess what? I'd run around 350 meters to this spot and then literally drop on the ground and start breathing heavily like a dog.

After 20 seconds I'd realize he is already anxiously waiting to see me and start running the next 350 meters left to him. So when I first could manage 2 laps. and then 3 laps, that was a victory. And when, after a month of running, I managed my first 5k charity run, I was thrilled. That was the biggest victory in life, and it remains the most exciting one so far (and remember, two marathons).

Why am I advising you in this book? Because I'm no champion, and no athlete. I'm a regular slightly overweight girl. I am quite a successful fashion business consultant in Russia, but nothing outstanding in relation to physical conditioning or aptitude. So I totally understand and feel what you feel and how you feel when you are about to start your first run.

You are scared it just won't work and you'll fail.

You are setting too ambitious of goals.

You are taking too long to prepare for a run.

Such are three most common problems once you make your mind to start running. And I can tell you, these were my problems right away. But, I can also tell you how to fix them.

First, don't postpone preparing for a run. All common prejudices about the right clothing and the right sneakers to wear, those don't matter for now. You are about to start running. You are about to run 1 kilometer, then 1 mile, then 2 kilometers, then 2 miles, etc. Believe me, none of those distances however challenging they might be, require special equipment. Regular sneakers you walk in, any yoga pants left from your childhood PE classes and any T-shirt you can find will do.

I've been running in winter in Moscow at 27 degrees below zero Celsius (-32 F) in a regular Uniqlo fleece jacket, two pairs of socks, average Nikes and woolen tights plus cheap Kaneji by Decathlon tights, a regular leopard (yeah, right) scarf and a woven hat. Guess what? Nothing happened.

I didn't get stripped in the middle of the street, and that's Russia where people tend to really worry about looks. So go ahead, put on whatever you can and go run, don't wait for better weather conditions or more free time. We are building a new habit here, and weather and stress are going to be imminently present at some stages.

Second, don't set too ambitious of goals. I once read a book about time management and procrastination. One wise thing it says is we tend to scare ourselves with too lofty of targets. The author gave an example of a person riding an elephant. Our elephant is our laziness and our habits to be not very active. So he was wondering, can the rider make the elephant follow his direction right away, from the very first time, when the rider is so small and the elephant is so big?

So he suggested not scaring and elephant and demanding too much of it, but moving step by step. If you have never been engaged in sports and you know your eating and sleeping habits are far from perfect, if you smoke and don't mind a glass of wine or a pint of beer here and there, don't start with long distances or durations for runs. The first step you should take is the following. Put on sneakers and running gear and get out in the street.

That's it. You must be shaking your head now. Really? How stupid that sounds. It actually is a very smart recommendation. Don't scare your elephant with long distances. Just wake up in the morning, get dressed for a run and get out in the street. Walk around the block and go home. You did it, you made your first step to being healthier, and it didn't hurt, did it? Right, so we can continue moving without putting our elephant away.

The next day you might actually feel like running

a little, but not more than a kilometer. Don't worry about time, it might take you anywhere from 8 to 10 minutes or even as little as 6 minutes if you are rushing it. But don't rush it.

Feel your body moving and follow your breathing. Try not to breathe heavily, it's two times inhaling and two times exhaling at every four steps you take, or two times inhaling and three times exhaling depending on whatever is better for you. Just make sure you don't run too hard. You can feel you are overdoing it when you hear your feet bumping the ground.

A real nice run is nice and easy, right? So you should try and step very light, as if you are running on air. For all of your early runs don't worry about pace or distances. Watch your step and your breath. Those are essential to keep you healthy and prevent any injuries that are likely if you push it too hard. Take your elephant step by step, increase not the distance but the time you run step by step.

Starting from 1 kilometer (or 10 minutes) and adding up a little time won't hurt you, I promise. Just don't increase the time or distance too drastically. For example running 1 kilometer, then 2 and the next day three kilometers isn't a way to build a sustainable habit. It's a way to make yourself sore and tired and hateful of running and runners. Running 1 kilometer, then 1.5 kilometers (or 1 mile) a couple times, then moving to 2 kilometers and sticking with this distance for two or three times and moving up to 3 the next week might be a better option. My suggested plan for your taking action and not scaring away your elephant would be as follows:

Days	Time	Distance
Week 1	Trying your elephant	
Monday	10 minutes	1-1.5 kilometers (depending on how far you can run in 10 minutes)
Tuesday	10 minutes	1-1.5 kilometers (depending on how far you can run in 10 minutes)
Wednesday	12 minutes	1 mile (1.6 kilometers)
Thursday	Cross-train	Do some basic exercises like squats and push ups and stretch

Friday	12 minutes	1 mile (1.6 kilometers)
Saturday	15 minutes	2 kilometers
Sunday	REST	REST
Week 2	Prepping your elephant	
Monday	12 minutes	1 mile (1.6 kilometers)
Tuesday	15 minutes	2-2.5 kilometers
Wednesday	20 minutes	3 kilometers
Thursday	Cross-train	Add +20% squats and pushups to what you did last week. Stretch!!!
Friday	22 minutes	2 miles (3.2 kilometers)
Saturday	25 minutes	3.5 kilometers
Sunday	REST	REST
Week 3	Working out your elephant	
Monday	15 minutes	2-2.5 kilometers
Tuesday	20 minutes	3 kilometers

Running Low And Slow

Wednesday	25 minutes	3.5 kilometers
Thursday	Cross-train	Add +20% squats and pushups to what you did last week. Stretch!
Friday	30 minutes	4-4.5 kilometers
Saturday	30 minutes	4-4.5 kilometers
Sunday	REST	REST
Week 4	Elephant breaking the limits	
Monday	20 minutes	3 kilometers
Tuesday	25 minutes	3.5 kilometers
Wednesday	30 minutes	4-4.5 kilometers
Thursday	Cross-train	Add +10% to what you did last week and... Stretch!!!
Friday	35 minutes	5 kilometers (a little over 3 miles)
Saturday	25 minutes	3.5 kilometers
Sunday	REST	REST

This is just a very vague example of how this might progress. You are an individual person, so you might be slower or faster than the given paces per kilometer. That is why mileage doesn't really matter. Just watch your running time.

By the end of the month you will be able to run for 35 minutes, and that is awesome. Another thing I might tell you about, that my coach wouldn't approve of. Walking is okay. I know every coach in the world says you should run non-stop. Right, if you are an athlete, or working to be one. We are running for pleasure, for better health and for happiness. So don't worry if at first you have to walk sometimes. Every time you run, try to stop less and ask yourself if you really need to stop.

If you do, that's okay, it's no big deal. The most important thing is you are staying out all this time. A whole 30 minutes a day you are working out. Your body sets the intensity, you set the pace and the rhythm. I only tell you should run for 30 minutes and you run as much of it as you can, then you walk for some time, and then get back to running. Just make sure not to stop without a reason.

I always stop because I'm lazy or because my brain tells my body to stop. I can confess to you I hardly every stop because I feel tired or injured or it's really hard to run. I stop because I decide to stop. I stopped during many races and I have yet to face running a marathon without stopping. I admit to you I'm not a perfect exemplary runner, but that's precisely why I'm writing this.

You win over yourself every time you choose to put on sneakers and get out to go run. You don't win when you cross the finish line first, you win when you cross it at any time, irrespective of when anybody does. So if you stop, it's okay, just make sure it doesn't disappoint you. Only you and your feelings matter. If it's too hard and your are too tired, walk some and then try to run some.

Once you question yourself, you will probably see that sometimes you stop because you are just merely bored with running, you feel sorry for yourself or there is something else bothering you which is not related to running. In this situation I can recommend you to have running buddies. By running buddies I'm not talking about people you'd like to run with if those people have been in running way longer and can already cover longer distances. By a running buddy I mean a beginner to running who is just starting too. Starting together would mean encouraging each other, not giving up in front of each other and not missing workouts, so as to not let each other down.

Daria Yadernaya

I started running when my partner in crime, Masha, suddenly got a crazy idea of running a half-marathon in Nice together. We had three months to prepare for these 21.1 kilometers in one of the most beautiful cities in the French Riviera. She wouldn't let me even consider this decision, and before I knew, we were already getting airplane tickets.

I was so nervous and my inner self was protesting so much that I made a mistake in the ticket and had to rebook it which cost me extra 50 Euros, and that was at the peak of the Ruble to Euro collapse when the ticket cost an average Moscow monthly salary. Our coach helped us build a program and so we started.

We would meet at the gym and run on treadmills together. Oh, yes, it was February so I wasn't even considering, at the time, running outside in Russian winter. That would come a year later with Paris marathon. God, I wanted to drop out every single workout we did, every 100 meters I'd think about it, then I'd look at Masha, envy her stamina and decide I'm not giving up unless she is giving up.

And so it went, she ran, and I ran too. We were both not particularly fast, but she was improving faster, and I tried to keep up. My motivation was low, hers was super high, she already saw us all young and sexy, tuned and fit, cruising La Promenade des Anglais. Meanwhile, I was more visualizing us all sweaty, red and puffy crawling the distance. She pushed me and dragged me and kicked my butt. I'm so grateful to her now that she did. Without her I'd never get to running at this scale, that is for sure.

Later I got more running buddies – the Moscow road runners club one of the most important benchmarks in this journey. It all started from a work contact with the founder of the club, Andrey, a month before my half-marathon in Nice. My first half-marathon ever. Six months before I could only do 700 meters and here I was preparing to knock down 21.1 kilometers.

He invited me into the community, and at first I was ashamed to take part in any of the group runs. I was too slow, too fat, too unfit. However, being part of the group chat, where everybody was always positive, always supportive, sharing their results and feelings. I finally decided I'd take part. We did a spectacular run from the Bolshoi Theater in Moscow through its heart to the Red Square and… well further it must have been beautiful too, but I had to drop out after 4 kilometers, that was too fast for me.

However, I did not give up and go home. I

continued my run the other way, at my pace, willing myself to knock out the 10 kilometers I planned for myself for that day. I tried running with them, and it was just too fast, but I stayed in the community, did a couple more runs with them. We did Moscow marathon together (well, I saw them at the starting line,) and some of us did Paris marathon too. And every day I get texts in this group chat and I feel I'm not alone.

I'm still way behind their paces and mileage in the group, but I'm staying. They are my running buddies, and I'm feeling part of the group, even though we can only start together. They will be running in Saint-Petersburg this summer, a marathon, I already did mine this year, but I'm so willing to cheer them on.

Thanks to them I believed the Moscow marathon was possible. Thanks to their friendly recommendations, and sometimes gentle kicks in the butt to start moving, I'm still on track. And planning to stay on track. I don't think about myself as a laggard of the group, rather the finalizing person, who makes sure the group is complete. Both the leaders, and the closing parties (that's me). And yes, some people in these 14 months I've been with the group have both joined the group, and left. Some of them just irritated by too many texts about runs they couldn't do or accomplish.

Running Low And Slow

My recent running buddy is my business assistant Sveta. She has been putting runs on my timetable for months before she decided to undertake running too. That was at the point where I was already on my way to training for the Paris marathon, so technically I was the more experienced buddy in this duet.

We would meet next to British Higher School of Art and Design in Moscow, next to Artplay cluster of art and architectural design, next to the Moscow river. She lives nearby, I work at British School as a lecturer (currently Head of Intensive Pro of Creative Entrepreneurship, a program on fashion startups and Head of Fashion Business program). We would meet and run 5 kilometers along the riverbank.

She started alone with less than one mile, claimed it almost killed her. The first time we ran together we chatted and she did 3 kilometers, almost 2 miles, in a week we brought it up to 5 kilometers and once even to 7 kilometers. All this was in about a month and a half, provided we ran together only once or twice a week because of my extensive travel.

Sveta believed I was helping her, in reality I was helping myself, sticking with running as often as possible, not giving up, building strength and stamina at a pace where I could also talk to her, my marathon pace that is. So we both helped each other, in our own way. She kept me practicing marathon pace and not skipping short and easy workouts, and I helped her chat away kilometers as she was getting her initiation into running.

All these and many other people I talked to and saw on social media helped me go on my journey, they encouraged me directly and indirectly every time I wanted to skip a run. The most important thing to remember, it's up to you and you only to decide how far you want to run and how long you want to run. The only basis for comparison is you today versus you yesterday. The only thing that matters you are working on it, you are moving toward your goal.

Don't try to increase mileage too fast, your elephant might get scared or, even worse, you might get injured. That happened to me two times in the 15 months I have been running, so believe me, I've been there and done that. Every time I tried to push my body past my limits, every time I rushed it or showed impatience, I paid the price.

I paid it before Nice, when I increased mileage too drastically and ended up with a twisted ankle and had to pause my training for 3 weeks. And losing 3 weeks out of the 12 I had to work for my first half-marathon not only took away from from my result, but most importantly from my self-confidence before the race. Pushing it too far after the Moscow marathon and trying to run a half-marathon in a week resulted in me not finishing the race because I fractured my foot.

I paid for it with two months of not running and then ,as December started, I was too lazy to get back into the routine. By the time I finally started in January, I had to start all over from the scratch and the Paris marathon was only three months away. Who knows how much better I could have done if I hadn't missed those three extra months of running.

After Paris, I kept running but was smart enough to pause my running for two weeks when seven days after the marathon once my foot started giving me signals of something is not right here. I paused my training just to avoid injury. Every time I believed I could push it higher and further and every time my body would react. So don't try and increase the intensity too rapidly even if it suddenly feels easy.

One of our famous Russian ultra-marathoners Eugenia Rumyantseva always posts her recommendations of at least a year of free running and getting into shape before even considering a serious long race, and she is right. I did it all wrong, because I was in a hurry to take part in races, get medals, share them on social media and prove my achievements to everyone around, even though it was mostly impressing myself. And the way I did it wasn't perfect, so I paid for it. Still, at this point in my life I believe I did it mostly right as I strongly needed the extra boost as I started running, and races gave me the boost that was needed.

3 WHY RACES ARE FUN

And we are coming upon the idea of actually taking part in a race. Why would I race? It's a competition and I'm just a beginner, and I'm not that fast a runner, or I wouldn't be able to maintain a long distance. All true, but...

Races have some fascinating aspects about them. They motivate you more than ever. Waking up every morning and going for a run is a challenge. Every time you do it, you win. However, finding reasons to run every morning is complicated. I don't know if I met many runners who would love to wake up early in the morning and go run. I met some, but they are few.

Most people are just like me. Every morning they wish they didn't have to wake up, get out of bed, put on the sneakers and run. First, running time is clearly subtracted from your sleep and even though we are all grown adults, we still go to bed as late as possible keeping ourselves busy with stupid stuff like surfing the web, exploring social media, watching TV or playing video games. So it's obviously hard to wake up one hour earlier at least to have time to get dressed, go run, come back, take a shower, change clothes, have breakfast and go to work.

Second, it just takes an effort to run so wanting to postpone or skip it is totally normal. Even when you start enjoying the actual process of running, making a decision to get out is still always a challenge.

Thirdly, every day you need to do more than the previous day, and this thought might also lead to your thoughts lingering on how hard it actually is. Races solve these problems to some extent. Yes, it's still hard to wake up, and you are still lazy, and you still don't want to do more, but there is a race coming. The date of a race is set, so you have no room for excuses. It's coming and you will have to get out and run the race on a set date.

Every missed workout is more suffering at the race day. A little accomplished every day provides for more pleasure and confidence during the competition. For me personally the main motivation was financial. I paid for the race. The first race we took part in was in Nice, and OMG it was expensive for me at a time.

The actual fee was only 25 Euros, but the flight was €500, the accommodation another €350, plus a visa and insurance and some money for taxis. Additionally, I had to buy expensive sneakers for another €140 (before I wore Oysho sneakers at €20 a pair), so my total price for running a Nice half-marathon €1000 plus money to have with me for food and shopping. At the time it was around what I made in a whole month, and my business was still highly unstable.

With me supporting Mum and investing everything I had in a business, this was quite an expense. So every day I didn't feel like running I'd remind myself of two things, Masha is waiting in the gym and God, I paid too much money to skip this now. As a result I was so nervous, especially when my ankle was hurt and I couldn't workout, that I got bronchitis exactly a week before the race. I had to go to Caspian Fashion Week on business and lecture there, which only made it worse. But, I was dead set on running in Nice and I did. I kept working out, kept taking care of my health, there was simply no way back.

The Moscow Marathon was not that expensive, but it was duty. My Moscow road runners invited me to run with them. It was my first race with the group, and I had to do well, i.e. in my case, finish the 42.2 kilometers (26.2 Miles). So whenever I'd feel like quitting, I'd think of the date approaching and my friends waiting for me at a starting line.

I'd sigh, curse, put on my sneakers and go run. I cursed and ran in Texas in suffocating heat and humidity. At times I ran at 3 am and at 4 am trying to avoid the sauna effect of the area. I ran in Greece in the mountains with no proper roads and the sun that was scalding you down to the bone. I got up at 4 am to finish my 30 kilometers by 8 when my Mum would wake up for breakfast. Trust me, at 4 am in Texas there is nobody running, as is in Greece before dawn. Oh, wait, in Greece I actually ran with mountain goats.

Races is what keeps me in shape, keeps me running not once or twice a week but following a certain program. Right now you do not even need a coach to have a simple program taking into account your running experience, age, weight and health condition. I'm using Nike Plus, but Runkeeper, Runtastic and Endomondo offer options for planning runs too.

They remind you of your runs, keep track of them, allow you to share them with friends. They motivate you and remind you of a race imminently coming, and this alone could get you going.

Running Low And Slow

Races are also a great place to make friends. Remember, running buddies? If nobody around you runs, they are too advanced or too focused on their runs; then a race is a great place to meet people just like you. The secret is you are not going to see many champions and winners, they will all start before you (and finish before you) so you won't see them at the starting or finishing line. The people that will be running with you or around you are those keeping up the same pace as you, so they might be your new friends at a race.

Races are long so exchanging a couple short phrases could set a basis for a further relationship and common runs. Races help you see how many people there are around who are just like you. When you run alone, or follow runners on social media, you might get confused and think you are the only slow person in the world, the only person who cannot run that far (underline whatever is relevant to you, that is). People who post runs would post brilliant results and show off perfect bodies and they are all such impeccable, ideal role models that sometimes make you feel inferior. Don't.

Most people are runners for pleasure and their results are very average. And even those people who do not run up to a certain standard set by somebody for their age or weight or health condition, they are still better than 99 per cent people on this planet. Running is becoming popular, that is true. However, even in the running countries like France or Italy, around 20 per cent of people run. That is they tend to run, go for a run sometimes, or just consider themselves runners. So still like around 80 per cent of the population do not run, and around 2/3 or them do not exercise in any way, shape or form.

So, getting out there means you already beat 75 per cent people on this planet just by merely making an effort. And you will see how many people like you there are around. They are all very normal healthy people who do not excel or set records. They do keep running and keep achieving new goals, getting better than they were a day before.

Races are also fun reason to travel. There are places on the planet you would never go visit, as you don't find a reason for it or it is too expensive or you don't have time, or many other reasons. I can tell you in 15 months I have been running, I found out more about my country than ever before. I travelled all sorts of towns and tiny villages as much as 300 kilometers away from Moscow (around 200 miles,) just for the sake of running there.

I saw beautiful cathedrals, charming rivers, fabulous lakes. I now know more of how an average

Russian lives and feels. I breathed the pure air of the village (me, a city girl,) and all because I made a choice to run there. I ran in places you'd never know or hear of. I know I haven't, and I'm Russian.

There was Bronnitsa, where I saw a beautiful lake and found out they host an internationally recognized triathlon there. Kubinka, where I discovered it has one of the biggest antique tank museums. And the cities of the Golden Ring. I hit Yaroslavl, Pereyaslavl, Rostov Veliky and Tutaev (ex Romanov-Borisoglebsk.) In a couple of days I'm headed to Kolomna to run an international Wings for Life race where the finish line represented by a catcher car is literally moving to catch you.

I went to Nice just to run and saw how beautiful the city is, and travelled to Monaco. In summer I wouldn't have gone as it is too expensive and in mid-season I wouldn't have gone as there is no point going to the sea unless it's summer, or there happens to be a half-marathon. I even ran on the track of Formula 1 in Sochi, how cool is that?

I studied the whole city of Paris during my 42.2 kilometer journey, and I'm up for more studies with the Ural trail run in three weeks, and a Golden Ring Ultra Trail in Suzdal mid-summer 2016. Would you travel to the Urals just for the sake of going? Me probably not, unless it's for work. But for a race… That is fun, I'm learning more about places, travelling to more places, and I'm doing it with a purpose, which is a very valid reason for visiting a new city, and getting new impressions out of it.

Races also give you medals. That might sound childish, but we all like to be praised and encouraged. Every race you finish, you get a medal. In 15 months I collected around 20 medals, and I am really proud of them. They are all hanging on the wall and looking at them, you might think I am actually a runner. And that matters a lot to me.

I am almost an athlete, only I am not, I am a very normal person, but the medals prove you have a whole right to be very proud of yourself. They are your trophies, you earned them, you sweated for them, you travelled for them. And they all keep their history even better than pictures in Instagram. And you don't have to scroll way down to find them.

They are witnesses of how you progressed, where you went and who you met. They show how many times you proved yourself you could do it, you could take another step and another one and cross the finish line. Running for medals might sound simplistic, but it's fun and motivating.

Running Low And Slow

And finally, the most common reason for quitting is actually boredom. Runners complain they get bored of running at the very beginning as they are too focused on how hard it is to move and they cannot think of anything else and they get bored and overwhelmed too fast. They try listening to music or watching movies when running on a treadmill, but it doesn't always work. My best suggestion for this is taking part in a race.

Once you are at a race, you won't need music or any other stimuli. You will be so immersed in the process, so many volunteers cheering you on, people running around you with their various sneakers, sports gear, faces and stories. The scenery will be constantly changing around you. And there will be music playing.

When running in Nice, I turned off my music as I was listening to the sea, the city and the seagulls. Believe me there is nothing like that in life. Once you feel it once, you will never be bored running again. And as soon as you start improving, you will be more and more focused on what's happening inside you than outside so you will be solving your inner problems. You will be busy planning your day and just relaxing and you will never be bored again. But the easiest way to achieve this is run a couple of races.

4 HOW TO CHOSE A RACE

So we decided you need to run a race. How do you choose a race? Obviously there are various factors to take into account.

1. distance to run
2. distance to where you live and how to get there
3. participation fee
4. accommodation or any other extra costs related
5. medical certificate required
6. past results required
7. medal or no medal
8. how old is the course
9. reviews of the course

So let's start with the distance to run. My suggestion always pick up a distance that is a next big challenge for you. I told you I started running from 700 meters, however by January I could half run, half walk 10 kilometers. So taking part in a 10k race wasn't exciting as I knew I could do it. The only question would be for me to do it faster. But, I wasn't excited about the fact I have to run fast. Secondly, travelling somewhere to run what I knew I could run wasn't fascinating. So we picked up a half-marathon. It was obviously impossible at this stage to tackle a marathon, but a half was enough of a challenge for somebody who could cover 10k with difficulty, but still possible to achieve.

Don't pick up a marathon if you have only run one half-marathon. You should run at least a couple of those and get better before you consider moving up. However, having 5k as your first race should be stimulating, if not, the maximum should be 10k. After doing a couple of those you might consider a half-marathon, but you should be in running for at least 6 months before your first half happens. And, you should be sure you are already able to cover at least 10k three months before the half marathon.

Many running schools prep you in 7 to 8 weeks, however I'd stress it's still for someone who already had at least some running experience or some fitness experience. If you never ever did anything sports related, this 7 to 8 weeks will just create an enormous shock on your body so you will finish your half but then feel put off of running or even worse, get injured. And we definitely don't want this. We want you a permanent champion with a wall full of medals.

The next question to consider is the financial one. And it's complex. First, how much are you willing to pay for a race? There are currently many races that are free of charge, organized by running schools or running clubs. So if you are just starting to run, you can try a couple of those runs. They might be more like fun runs, without a medal or a bib to time your run, but they will create crowds of people and volunteers that is a great motivation and encouragement.

If you are willing to pay the race, pay attention to some facts. First, most race fees are non-refundable. If you are not sure you are going to run, you might just waste money. Some races have an extra fee for insurance that promised you your money back if you don't run, but it means extra €8 to €10 for a European race.

Second, most races have extras that you might want to consider. I always pay in advance for having my medal engraved. It's great to have your name and time engraved on your medal and paying in advance is cheaper and it saves you time in the queues right after the race. Many races have pasta parties or guided tours of the city included for free or for a small fee, so you might also want to consider those.

Some races in Europe automatically include a branded T-shirt, others don't and you might be willing to pay for it to have a collection of T-shirts of cities you ran in and races you finished. By the way, Russian practice is you first get a T-shirt and then you run. In Paris, however, you have to finish the race as the T-shirt says Marathon Finisher in Paris. Anyway, Amsterdam for instance gives a T-shirt for free if you pay a marathon fee, but requires you to pay another €25 if you are running a half-marathon but still want to get a T-shirt.

Another part of the financial side is how much the total expense is going to be. A race might be not expensive. Barcelona and Nice are all around €25, for instance, races in Russia are €10 to €15 on the average, however for me to fly to Barcelona and stay there at a hotel would result in a completely different cost, just as Nice and Paris do.

So some more expensive races in my area might be actually more affordable for me, and vice versa. Like a fee to Run in Lyon or Reims would be €15 to €25, but for me to fly there from Moscow is a fortune unless I figure out trains. And even if I do, it's then time consuming which would mean taking a longer vacation to run this race, which again is money.

The next issue to consider is a medical certificate. In some races it is enough to sign a waiver, and you are free to go. In other races you need to produce a valid medical certificate, issued no more than 6 months before the race, allowing you to take part in a race. Be careful about the certificate and look at the sample form the race organizers provide to avoid any problems.

Some organizers require the distance allowed to be set in the medical certificate, so it should say you are able to run 10k/ half-marathon/marathon. Others would be happy with a certification you have no health issues preventing you from running. Pay attention to the language of the certificate, e.g. Paris strongly recommends certificates in French, and Nice was okay with an English certificate. Both are a nightmare to get in Moscow, and very expensive too, see above on extra costs.

Make sure you have both a copy of a certificate and an original when headed to the race. When you produce only an original, the organizing company takes it, and you will need to undergo the process to get a new one again every time you need to sign up for a new race. If you have a copy, they will check it against the original and take just the copy. Currently many Russian races have a copying machine next to the doors ready for free copying, however in Nice or Paris I didn't notice anything like that.

Some races are limited in terms of beginner runners. New York City Marathon is one of the best known marathons of the world, and one of the most difficult to get into. Unless you can produce a very good result for the past year, it's very difficult to qualify. They do have a lottery though, so you could win slots. Another way is to travel via a travel agency that holds slots, but as you might have guessed it is also going to cost a small fortune.

You results also determine the spot you get in the starting clusters too. The better your results, the earlier you start a race. The bib counts your individual time as soon as you cross the starting line, so don't worry about times. Let the fast and the daring start first, you will keep yourself from being overtaken in the crowd of crazy fast runners. Let them all pass and here comes your nice and easy jog with taking pictures and enjoying life.

Not all races give out medals at the end. For beginners, and not even accomplished runners, getting a medal is important. It shows you won, you finished, you smashed it. So pay attention to the whether a race has medals for everybody. We are collecting our wins and our memories, so we don't want to miss out.

How old is the course?

This question might seem a little off and a little careless in terms of the serious things we have discusses. However, it matters. If the race has existed for a long time, the distance is already checked by many runners and all possible complications are already numbered and counted. Water and food will be right where needed and in right amounts. There will be enough volunteers, there will be no wholes on the road and the course is going to match the mileage. Overall, the organization is going to be way better.

Now that running is booming, many companies are setting up their own runs. The first time is never perfect. They lack water and food, sometimes they lack volunteers, the route is far from perfect, the weather is unpredictable, T-shirts look crappy, and many other things. After being in the running world for some time you might find it entertaining and adventurous to take part in those races, however, that is not the best one to start with.

I took part in a couple of races with no T-shirts, no medals, no water (just hot tea,) no volunteers, no automated timing for the race, no place to change (a tent set on the cold ground at below zero doesn't count), and it's only fun when it's your 10th race or so. First races need to be perfect, they build a sound foundation for your enjoyment to run and the competition.

Finally, try and read the reviews of the course. All courses are different not only in distance but in surface. Different elevation, different surface (road or trail,) weather changes. Those all affect how you run. I was choosing a marathon between an Authentic Marathon in Athens, Marathon in Rome and Paris Marathon.

Rome is a city founded on the seven hills, and that might give you a hint of why I didn't choose it. Athens is a marathon where you run almost 20 kilometers down to the sea level and then 20 kilometers up back to Athens. Temperatures are high and the elevation changes intimidating. Paris is mostly flat and includes two forests that guarantees shadow and nice cool air to breathe. Nice was 70 per cent seaside and very flat, also running to the airport and back. Running next to the planes taking off and landing was kind of cool.

Being ready for what you are going to see on the course is important. It might be cold, might be rainy, the surface might be far from perfect, hills might be high. This all can affect your results and you might be really upset if you did better at workouts, in different conditions.

Another important thing is how the course is built in terms of entertainment. I ran one lap marathons, and that was cool, and I ran a 5-lapse half-marathons, and that was really getting on nerves. Having to run the same place for five times again and again, especially knowing what exactly is waiting for me and exactly how hard this might be.

5 WHY LOSING A RACE IS WINNING A RACE

Some of my friends think it's really depressing if they cannot finish among the top finishers of the race. They try to pass on competitions as they feel like they are losing it. I think I'm the best person to tell you about it. I normally finish closer to the last ones than to the first ones, so I know exactly how it feels to be doubting if there is anybody running behind you or if you might be the last person finishing the race.

I can confess to you that I felt depressed my early races when I did worse than I expected, and every single race I had in my first 10 months of running I did worse than expected. I was well prepared and confident I could do better and I didn't. Masha passed me by 10 to 12 minutes at all times, even though I believed we underwent the same training. Yet she got so strong-willed at races she never gave up and just went for her objective. I did so well at trainings and regular runs, but at races I felt I was losing it, so I lost it. Predominantly losing it to myself.

I was so upset I was considering giving up racing even though all those people volunteering at races cheered me up and stayed with me while I ran (or walked) and said nice encouraging things to me. So at some point I realized I need to stop worrying about it. I ran for myself, my results were for myself. The reason I couldn't achieve better results was my mind blocked me from doing it.

I didn't enjoy what I did. In three months I went to a half-marathon, and in another three I knocked out another half-marathon 12 minutes faster than the first one. After another two months, another one fell 12 minutes faster than the previous one. In nine months from the start I ran a marathon.

In winter I even mastered winter running and did a sub-zero half-marathon twice. Then I ran another marathon in Paris. These were my achievements, but I focused on how many people were faster than me, not how many people ran with me, how many finished (me among them) or how many did not run at all.

At some point I started realizing how many precious moments I was depriving myself of. I loved travelling, loved finishing, loved getting medals, loved sharing all about it on Facebook and Instagram. I still do. And getting encouragement on social media is important for me and it keeps me going. But I was always ashamed of my result. Until one moment, when I was picking up my race number and my bib in Paris, I picked up a couple of running magazines that were lying there. I took a bus home and while on the bus I was reading.

The Runners World magazine published an article about a woman who won a Paris marathon in 2014. She won it, the article declared. Did she come first? Nope. Regina, 52 years old, came last in 2014 at the Paris marathon. She won it, she smashed it. The article dwelled on how she felt when she ran and when she realized she was the last one. She shared how touched she was when volunteers were shouting to her "Go Regina, Go!" when she was plodding towards the finish line.

Nobody went away, everybody stayed and waited will she won the race. 6 hours 34 minutes after she started, she won. No, she never even saw the runners with the top times. The "winner" started the race at 8:45, her last cluster (just like mine in 2016) started at 10:50. The winner in 2014 finished at something like 2:05. The best time was a little slower in 2016. Kenenisa Bekele crossed the finish line at 10:50 or around so in 2014 in Paris when Regina hadn't even run her first 5 k.

By the time she finished the winner might have had food, taken a shower and a nap. But what does it matter? She won it just the same way as the more venerable athletes did. She conquered herself, just as they did. She made herself finish, just as they did. She was a star of the day, as everybody was. Perhaps more-so.

My year (2016) had 57 thousand registrations. Only 43000 of those even showed up to run, and around 40 thousand finished. Women represent only 25 per cent of those registered. This year had 40 thousand winners, and I was among them. In fact I was among the way fewer women who dared to even try to run the Paris marathon. The planet is inhabited by billions of people, but most of them never ran and never will.

I did it, I ran a marathon and I had a will to finish. It doesn't matter there were only 200 people behind me. The day before the race I learned the truth. When I had been reading about Regina, I was crying. I was proud of her, and proud of me ever since. My times don't matter, I just finished. My time was perfect, it was mine.

Being at the end is flattering too. It's hard for you, everybody around sees it and understands. You are not a professional athlete who has all the time in the world and money from sponsors to prepare.

Running Low And Slow

You are a regular person, with personal life and work load to handle. Things to do in life. Running is only part of your life, the part you cherish and try to develop, but obviously not at the expense of other parts of your life.

You win by merely showing up at the starting line, you win twice by crossing the finish line. You win every day by getting out to run, by taking every next step and pushing yourself to longer distances or faster paces. You are better than you were yesterday, and this doesn't depend on the measurement of your results getting better.

At some point I had to admit I'm not going to just get faster for a marathon, unless I go back to my 5k's and work on getting faster at shorter distances. I admit I'll never be super fast but I can go a little faster. And I need to step backwards and working on my shorter distances. I need to run a half marathon without walking or stopping first, before I look at another marathon. But even with these imperfections I have and admit, I still finished marathons. Twice.

I will cherish this as an achievement for life. I know I will run again, a marathon each year sounds nice, but I'm not going to bet on it. We will see how I feel. And how strong the feeling will be to experience the glory of a marathon again. The Nike

Plus app has a greatest encouragement ever for the day of the race. It says. This morning you wake up a runner and when you go to bed, you'll be a marathoner.

I want to race more, and I will. It's fun, adventure and travel. It is everything I love in life. And I love me, crossing the finish line, me getting the medal and me posting it on Instagram. One of the encouraging posters on the course in Saint-Petersburg where I ran 10k said "Pain is temporary and the glory of Instagram is forever!" That's hilarious, but this works for them, and if it works for you too, there is nothing wrong with it.

Whatever, if it makes you happy and doesn't hurt anybody around is a good positive thing. Racing is fun, it helps you stay healthy and happy, meet new friends and feel you are not alone. You get feel how many people run with you, irrespective of how fast and fit you are. And even if you happen to be the last one to finish, it's just a symbol of your greatest victory. It's your victory over yourself and billions of people who never bothered to move their selves off the couch to go and try to run.

You are healthier, happier, more wholesome and fulfilled every day you run. This depends only on putting the sneakers on and getting out there, not on the distances you covered or hours you spent running. Medals, maybe, a little bit. LOL, just joking (kind of,) but I'll bet you that you'll love having medals too.

We are just people and people like toys and treasures. Medals are both. They remind us of the most precious treasure we have, ourselves. With our complex feelings and inner struggles, where we win and win all over again, pushing ourselves higher, better, faster.

Moving is life, and you are moving ahead faster than many, and most importantly, faster than you yesterday. You definitely win, so my congratulations on the victory and many more to go.

Congratulations!!!

PS

I've hereby shared my own experience of running and getting started as a runner, my feelings, emotions and sensations of my journey through the fascinating world of running and becoming a race-participant. All recommendations I give are purely experience-based and are in no way marketed or promoted by any companies or brands I name in my book. None of them sponsored me to mention them or promote them and I'm not an adept of any of the leading sports brands like Nike, Adidas, Puma, Mizuno or Decathlon. I combine them depending on my goals and weather conditions. I mention the Nike plus app too among other apps by other companies but I personally prefer the Nike as it seems the most convenient for a beginner runner and it has no relation or affiliation to Nike as it is. All races I named are those I picked myself, paid myself and in no way received reimbursement from the, so they are all just my experience.

If you want to share you running experience, share with me and my followers different races you took part in or are planning to run, trail runs, mountain running etc. please don't hesitate to email me at d.yadernaya@gmail.com

ABOUT THE AUTHOR

Daria Yadernaya is a Moscow-based fashion business consultant, founder and owner of a fashion think-tank Y Consulting, Head of Educational Programs of Fashion Business and Creative Entrepreneurship: how to found a fashion startup and a business coach on building startups in fashion industry in Russia and the CIS countries